Made in the USA
Columbia, SC
02 May 2023

16023138R00070